CONDOM SENSE

A GUIDE TO SEXUAL SURVIVAL IN THE NEW MILLENNIUM

M. MONICA SWEENEY, MD, MPH
RITA KIRWAN GRISMAN

LANTERN BOOKS • NEW YORK
A DIVISION OF BOOKLIGHT INC.

2005
Lantern Books
One Union Square West, Suite 201
New York, NY 10003

Printed in the United States of America

"Protecting the Planet" photograph by Joseph Sweeney

Library of Congress Cataloging-in-Publication Data

Sweeney, M. Monica
Condom sense : a guide to sexual survival in the new millennium / by M. Monica Sweeney, Rita Kirwan Grisman.
p. ; cm.
Includes bibliographical references.
ISBN 1-59056-077-9 (alk. paper)
1. AIDS (Disease)—United States—Prevention. 2. HIV infections—United States—Prevention. 3. Condoms—United States. 4. Safe sex in AIDS prevention—United States. I. Grisman, Rita Kirwan. II. Title.
[DNLM: 1. HIV Infections—prevention & control—Popular Works. 2. Condoms—utilization—Popular Works. 3. Safe Sex—Popular Works. WC 503.6 S974c 2005]
RA643.83.S94 2005
362.196'9792—dc22
2004020873

Lantern Books has elected to print this title on New Leaf Eco Offset, a 100% post-consumer recycled paper, processed chlorine-free. As a result, we have saved the following resources.

7 trees, 1,582 gallons of water, 346 lbs of solid waste, 3 million BTUs energy,
0.0 years of electricity required by the average US home, 585 lbs greenhouse gases,
511 miles traveled in the average American car, 1 lb of air emissions
(HAPs, VOCs, TRSs combined), 14 lbs of hazardous effluent (BODs, TSSs, CODs, AOXs)

As part of Lantern Books' commitment to the environment we have joined the Green Press Initiative, a nonprofit organization supporting publishers in using fiber that is not sourced from ancient or endangered forests. For more information, visit www.greenpressinitiative.org.

THIS BOOK IS DEDICATED TO EVERYONE WHO UNDERSTANDS, OR WHO WANTS TO UNDERSTAND, THAT WE CAN NEVER TREAT OUR WAY OUT OF THE AIDS PANDEMIC, AND THAT THE BEST TREATMENT FOR ANY DISEASE IS NOT GETTING IT.

ACKNOWLEDGMENTS

To my best friend and life's partner, Joseph Lee Sweeney, without whose support this book, like all my projects, could not have happened. When the computer was down, you fixed it; when my spirit was down, you lifted it. For everything, always, thank you! Thanks to my children and grandchildren, for when I missed special family times and you understood. Thanks to Evelyn and Everett Ortner for the clippings, the calls, and the collations; you are friends indeed. And to Norris Chumley for introducing us to Gene Gollogly, who was able to get behind our mission.

—M.M.S.

Thank you, my dear Arnold, for your patience and punctuation. To the Albany Medical College, Division of HIV Medicine, and to Cathryn Corlew, our gratitude.

—R.K.G.

TABLE OF CONTENTS

CHAPTER ONE

WHY I WROTE THIS BOOK

47,000,000 infected, 0 cured

Sometime in the '80s, I got into an elevator that a New York bicycle messenger was exiting. I suspect it was he who had scratched the heartfelt graffiti on one elevator wall: "Love Makes You Crazy."

That bicycle messenger knew what he was writing about. His message wakes me up and weighs me down whenever I prepare one of my lectures on what has become my life's mission: to educate everybody about the perils of sexually transmitted diseases, with unrelenting emphasis on AIDS, because, simply put, AIDS kills you.

I'm all in favor of love, and of sex, for that matter—perhaps too much in favor of it—but as a doctor I know that the thrill of sex, no matter how crazy in love the lovers, must be accompanied by protection. The condom—historically a way to avoid pregnancy, a sort of swaggering symbol for the young, or the source of speechless embarrassment for people in the throes of first love, a source of jokes or giggles or guffaws—is an item no one can afford to dismiss, because a condom can keep you from dying.

We are over twenty years into the AIDS pandemic, and the focus is still on treatment. The CDC has finally recommended a program designed to cut HIV infection from 40,000 new cases a year to 20,000 a year. The plan has met with some resistance from AIDS activists who suggest that focusing the prevention message on those people already infected might lead to greater stigmatization. In my view, the list of those at risk is ever expanding, so everyone needs to know their HIV status. One organization out of San Francisco says it best, in their name and their mission, "HIV Stops With Me."

Yet most of the available money is spent on treatment. What a pity, since the way to prevent sexual transmission of the virus is so simple:

Condoms.

(Addicts' needle-sharing is another way to transmit the AIDS virus. It is another terrible, far-reaching problem, but one I'm not dealing with here, right now).

The health of the world depends on condoms, not

abstinence. Abstinence is a statistically 100 percent perfect solution to the prevention of sexual transmission of AIDS, but it is also, among most of the population, a fantasy. Sadly, now in greater numbers than ever, the world's populations are behaving in increasingly dangerous and reckless ways when it comes to sex.

Teenagers, both male and female, are making themselves available to older men. These kids are called sex workers, and they show up on the streets of cities, not necessarily in bad neighborhoods or on back streets, but in places where they can be spotted as willing partners. In return for sex, they get money for the favored object of the day: jeans, watches, video equipment, audio equipment, CDs, computer games. The sex is fast, anonymous, and unprotected, murderously impersonal to the participants, who go on their way and pass the disease to their unsuspecting partners. The clients don't take responsibility, and the kids think they're immortal. Other people get AIDS; never the young, the strong, the beautiful.

The other trend is sex for sport. It's the return of the kind of sex that was rampant at the beginning of the AIDS pandemic, when men in large cities went to bath houses and sex clubs for sex. Of course, heterosexuals are no strangers to sex for sport. Fortunately, places like

Plato's Retreat (a notorious sexual playground in New York City) have been closed. But clubs featuring lap dancing still flourish, and the dancing bears no resemblance to the waltz.

Some men, dazzled by the possibility of sex as a contact sport, are taking sex to a new low. They frequent places called glory holes, which are set up so that the sexual partners never see one another eye to eye. The sex is purely mechanical and literally faceless. It might as well be robotic, except that robots can't catch STDs or pass them on.

And, sadly, irresponsible behavior isn't limited to the young. As the United States ages, senior citizens are contracting the disease they thought was the province of other age groups, other cultures. It's happening particularly in the United States because of our huge population of aging, having-it-all Baby Boomers—who are now acquiring something they do *not* want.

There are, of course, treatments that help forestall some of the misery that comes with AIDS, and help to prolong life. But these treatments carry a financial and emotional cost that is too high for most people to bear. They are certainly no cure for a pandemic that claims thousands of lives every year.

I wrote this book to convince you to take condoms

seriously and to help you take responsibility for your love life, your sex life, your secret life. I intend to help allay any anxiety or embarrassment about the use of condoms, to inform you of options if you discover you've gotten the virus, and to make it crystal clear that *AIDS doesn't happen to someone else.*

Nobody can ever be too informed about condoms, or about the irrevocable pain their use prevents.

You can't bring back the dead.

And, for all those guys who posture and rant about the pleasure that condoms deprive them of, I have this question: have you ever had an orgasm worth dying for?

This book is for all of you who answered, *"No."*

CHAPTER TWO

SELF-ASSESSMENT

47,000,000 infected, 0 cured

W hen, and why, do you think you need to use a condom? This could be the most important test you ever take. Answers are at the end.

TRUE   FALSE

1. **The following diseases can be transmitted through sexual activity.**

		TRUE	FALSE
a)	Hepatitis A	❏	❏
b)	Hepatitis B	❏	❏
c)	Syphilis	❏	❏
d)	Gonorrhea	❏	❏
e)	Monilia (yeast)	❏	❏
f)	Chlamydia	❏	❏

	TRUE	FALSE
g) Chancroid	❏	❏
h) HIV	❏	❏
i) Human papillomavirus (HPV, genital warts)	❏	❏
j) Hepatitis C	❏	❏
k) Lice or nits (Pediculus pubis)	❏	❏
l) Herpes Simplex virus (HSV-1, HSV-2)	❏	❏
m) Trichomoniasis	❏	❏

2. **The following diseases can be cured.**

	TRUE	FALSE
a) Hepatitis A	❏	❏
b) Hepatitis B	❏	❏
c) Syphilis	❏	❏
d) Gonorrhea	❏	❏
e) Monilia	❏	❏
f) Chlamydia	❏	❏
g) Chancroid	❏	❏
h) HIV	❏	❏
i) Human papillomavirus	❏	❏
j) Hepatitis C	❏	❏
k) Lice	❏	❏
l) Herpes	❏	❏
m) Trichomoniasis	❏	❏

		TRUE	FALSE

3. If a potential sexual partner shows you the results of his/her negative HIV test done just four days ago, you can forget about using condoms.   ❑   ❑

4. You are very careful about choosing a sexual partner. Your partner's HIV test is negative, and his or her sex organs appear healthy. You can forget about using condoms.   ❑   ❑

5. You are HIV-positive. You've finally met an HIV-positive partner and you two have decided to have sex. You can forget about using condoms.   ❑   ❑

6. Your partner, who has been incarcerated for the past seven months, is coming home. You are eight months pregnant. You can forget about using condoms.   ❑   ❑

	TRUE	FALSE
7. The following body fluids may contain HIV.		
a) Saliva	❑	❑
b) Urine	❑	❑
c) Tears	❑	❑
d) Sweat	❑	❑
e) Vaginal secretions	❑	❑
f) Menstrual blood	❑	❑
g) Breast milk	❑	❑
h) Semen ("cum")	❑	❑
i) All of the above	❑	❑
j) None of the above when the viral load is undetectable	❑	❑
8. Whether you use condoms or not, everyone who has sex should get an HIV test every three months.	❑	❑
9. Oral sex is not really sex and therefore does not carry any risk for spreading HIV or other STDs.	❑	❑
10. Women who have sex with women don't have to worry about HIV and other STDs.	❑	❑

		TRUE	FALSE
11.	Receptive anal intercourse is the riskiest sexual act for transmission of HIV, and the only sex act for which a condom must be used at all times.	❏	❏
12.	My sexual partner is HIV-positive and I am HIV-negative. His viral load is undetectable. He doesn't have to wear a condom.	❏	❏
13.	I don't know why everyone still gets so excited about becoming HIV-positive. It's just like any other chronic disease.	❏	❏
14.	There is a "morning-after pill" that will protect you from getting HIV if you've had risky sexual behavior the night before.	❏	❏
15.	If an HIV-positive woman is pregnant and takes her medication (antiretrovirals), her baby will definitely not be born HIV-positive.	❏	❏

Answers to Self-Assessment

1.   **a) through m) are all true.**
     All can be transmitted sexually, though it also is pos-
     sible to contract Hepatitis A, monilia (yeast infection),
     or lice without being sexually active.

2.   a) **True.**
         Hepatitis A is a self-limiting disease and does not
         become chronic or cause liver failure like hepatitis B
         and C.
     b) **False.**
     c) **True.**
     d) **True.**
     e) **True.**
     f) **True.**
         Chlamydia is curable but can cause irreversible dam-
         age; though often present without symptoms in both
         men and women, it is the most common cause of steril-
         ity in women. Chlamydia can also cause chronic pelvic
         pain, referred to as PID (pelvic inflammatory disease).
     g) **True.**
     h) **False.**
         The purpose of this book is to let everyone know that
         HIV leads to AIDS, which is both deadly and incurable,
         with over 47,000,000 people infected and zero cured.
     i) **False.**
         HPV, human papillomavirus, can take up to one year
         from the time of contact with an infected person for

warts to develop. There is a strong association between HPV and cervical cancer. Condoms don't provide complete protection against HPV, just the best available if you have sex.

j)   **False.**
k)   **True.**
l)   **False.**
m)   **True.**

Trichomoniasis is curable but often requires repeated treatment before it is eradicated.

3.   **False.**

Even a negative HIV test does not prove the bearer is negative. He or she could be in the window period—the time after infection before the antibody blood test becomes positive.

4.   **False.**

As stated above, HPV, human papillomavirus, can take up to one year from the time of contact with an infected person for warts to develop.

5.   **False.**

Even if two people are HIV-positive, they should use condoms. The exact extent to which cross and super infection happens is still under debate. However, becoming infected with a different, more potent or resistant virus is well documented, not only with HIV strains but also with other STDS. Your virus may be more sensitive to treatment than your partner's.

6.   **False.**
     Prisons are feeding grounds for HIV, since condoms are often not available and prisoners are often willing as well as unwilling sexual partners.

7.   **True.**
     All of the listed fluids (a through h) can contain the virus even when the viral load is undetectable in serum.

8.   **False.**
     Everyone does not need an HIV test every three months. We need to know our status and then avoid behaviors that put us at risk. The test is not protective.

9.   **False.**
     Whether or not you think it's "real sex," oral sex puts you at real risk for STDs, including HIV.

10. **False.**
     Although rare, transmission of HIV can occur between women.

11. **False.**
     Although anal sex carries the greatest risk of transmis- sion of HIV, vaginal and oral sex also carry risk, and

condoms should always be used. For oral sex per-
formed on women, use a dental dam, or in a pinch
plastic wrap can be protective. Some people even split
open an unlubricated condom to serve as protection
during oral sex.

12.   **False.**
The lower the viral load, the less likely the transmission. However, even when the virus is undetectable in
serum, it is still detectable in semen and vaginal fluids.

13.   **False.**
AIDS is not just like other chronic diseases. AIDS is a
chronic disease that results in many other chronic diseases, one of which will probably kill you.

14.   **False.**
The practice of taking one pill (antiretroviral) after
risky sexual behavior is not protective against becoming infected with HIV. Under the supervision of an
HIV/AIDS expert, a health care worker can treat those
exposed to infection to decrease the risk of serocon-
version (becoming HIV-positive).

15.   **False.**
A pregnant woman can decrease, but not eliminate, the
risk of her unborn child being HIV-positive if she takes
the antiretrovirals while pregnant.

CHAPTER THREE

AIDS: A DEADLY DISEASE
AND GETTING DEADLIER

47,000,000 infected, 0 cured

S preading faster than the Black Death (which took more than three centuries to kill 137 million people) and more deadly than the influenza pandemic of 1918 (which killed more people than World War I, between 20 and 40 million), AIDS is the fastest-growing and most extensive plague in human history. There are 47 million infected so far, and the numbers are rising. Meanwhile, this disease, so far, shows no sign of ending.

AIDS is short for Acquired Immune Deficiency Syndrome. That means the body's defenses against illness are too weakened to counter all kinds of diseases, so infections occur that don't usually occur in people with healthy immune systems. These infections are called "opportunistic." The carriers of the virus are prey to every illness imaginable. Even the common cold becomes threatening.

The media images that portray people living with AIDS as lively and robust don't reflect the reality of life with the disease. Even the AIDS-infected who are undergoing the newest treatments don't live life feeling well or functioning fully. Magic Johnson is not a realistic poster boy for this disease. Most people don't start out with his extraordinary health advantages, or his resources.

Early in the course of AIDS the infected person has fevers, swollen glands, night sweats, weight loss, chills, and weakness. Sometimes AIDS first presents as tuberculosis. The end stages are marked by cancer of the lymph glands, Kaposi's Sarcoma (just two of an assortment of cancer possibilities), meningitis, dementia.

AIDS is caused by a virus called Human Immunodeficiency Virus (HIV). Almost everybody with HIV gets AIDS. No one with AIDS is ever cured.

There is some research indicating that HIV spread from monkeys to humans between 1926 and 1946. Even more recent research shows that HIV probably jumped from chimpanzees to humans in 1675, but didn't settle in as a strain with epidemic possibilities until 1930. Researchers now say the first proven AIDS death in the world was in the Congo in 1959. This early AIDS case was identified by researchers who went back and tested blood samples, saved from 1959, from patients who died of mysterious diseases.

In 1978, a sickness started showing up in gay men in the U. S. and Sweden, and among heterosexuals in Haiti and Tanzania, that would later be identified as AIDS.

In 1981 the *New York Times* published its first article on AIDS, characterizing the disease as a rare cancer that had been seen in 41 homosexuals. And the CDC started noticing an alarming rate of another rare cancer, Kaposi's Sarcoma, showing up in gay men who were otherwise healthy. The disease was first called "gay cancer," then renamed GRID, an acronym for "gay-related immune deficiency."

In that same year, 1981, the illness and fatalities from this mysterious new disease began their inexorable rise.

In the United States alone . . .

- In 1981, 422 AIDS cases were diagnosed, and 159 people died of AIDS.
- In 1982, the total rose to 1,614 AIDS cases and 619 deaths.
- In 1983, the total rose to 4,749 AIDS cases and 2,122 deaths.

- In 1984, the total rose to 11,055 AIDS cases and 5,620 deaths.
- In 1985, the total rose to 22,996 AIDS cases and 12,592 deaths.
- In 1986, the total rose to 42,255 AIDS cases and 22,669 deaths.
- In 1987, the total rose to 71,176 AIDS cases and 41,027 deaths.
- In 1988, the total rose to 106,994 AIDS cases and 62,100 deaths.
- In 1989, the total rose to 149,902 AIDS cases and 89,817 deaths.
- In 1990, the total rose to 198,466 AIDS cases and 121,250 deaths.
- In 1991, the total rose to 257,750 AIDS cases and 157,637 deaths.
- In 1992, the total rose to 335,211 AIDS cases and 198,322 deaths.
- In 1993, the total rose to 422,887 AIDS cases and 241,787 deaths.
- In 1994, the total rose to 479,756 AIDS cases and 288,590 deaths.
- In 1995, the total rose to 534,806 AIDS cases and 332,249 deaths.

- In 1996, the total rose to 548,102 AIDS cases and 343,000 deaths.
- In 1997, the total rose to 548,102 AIDS cases and 364,999 deaths.
- In 1998, the total rose to 665,357 AIDS cases and 405,028 deaths.
- In 1999, the total rose to 706,028 AIDS cases and 418,200 deaths.
- In 2000, the total rose to 774,467 cases and 448,060 deaths.
- In 2001, the total rose to 807,071 AIDS cases and 462,653 deaths.
- In 2002, the total rose to 980,000 AIDS cases and 501,669 deaths.

In 2002, there were approximately 1.2 million people infected with HIV, with roughly 200,000 of these unaware that they were infected, just in the United States.*

Worldwide, approximately 47 million are currently infected. As of 2001, there were 15 million children who had been orphaned by AIDS worldwide, which equals the number of children under the age of five in the entire United States.

---

* All numbers for HIV/AIDS and AIDS deaths are cumulative.

The catastrophic expansion of this plague, though preventable, continues because of denial, irresponsibility, selfishness, immorality, politics, negligence, hopelessness, arrogance, indifference, laziness, and plain old stupidity. As medical science helps people with AIDS feel better longer, some have sex while they are contagious. One third of the HIV-infected population knows it's infected but continues to have unprotected sex. Another 25 percent of those infected with HIV don't realize they're infected and unknowingly spread the virus. These are two of the groups on which the CDC has begun to focus its efforts to decrease the spread of HIV. (Chapters such as "The Politics of Condoms" will talk more about some of the other problems I've mentioned above.)

It's been a long road and slow going.

Progress has been made with new drugs and treatments. Everybody knows something about the "cocktail" that forestalls the disease but doesn't cure it. The cost for a one-year regimen is between $12,000 and $15,000, and increasing all the time. The cost of treatment has created a financial crisis, so that currently in 10 U.S. states and most of the rest of the developing world, people are desperately waiting for funding for AIDS drugs.

We are spending millions and millions on a vaccine

to prevent this plague—a vaccine that might work for a while, but will not be clever enough to conquer the Human Immunodeficiency Virus, which will eventually mutate just when it seems like the AIDS battle has been won. There is a good reason that a vaccine hasn't been developed for the common cold, and that to be pro-tected from the flu viruses you have to have annual immunizations: viruses mutate, and what once worked stops working. The Human Immunodeficiency Virus is an even greater challenge.

Viewed by some as another quick fix on the horizon is the promise of a microbicide. A microbicide, like the spermicides you may be familiar with, is a substance, like a gel or cream, applied to reduce the transmission of the disease during sex. Zeda Rosenberg, CEO of the International Partnership for Microbicides, which is calling for a $1 billion microbicide research project, told the *San Francisco Chronicle* in July 2004 that although six microbicides are slated to begin clinical trials, she does not expect an effective one to be avail-able for five to seven years.

The cost of a package of a dozen condoms is about $12.00 ($8.00/dozen on the internet). You do the math for your yearly condom expense, based on your life, your lifestyle, your fun quotient.

So where does that leave us? Where we started: with condoms to prevent the sexual transmission of AIDS.

Keep reading.

CHAPTER FOUR

WHO GETS INFECTED WITH AIDS, AND HOW?

47,000,000 infected, 0 cured

A t first the AIDS plague appeared to be limited to the homosexual community, with the exception of blood transfusion recipients who received infected blood and blood products—a form of transmission that is now rare. The virus was quickly transmitted to the heterosexual community. Women are now one of the fastest-growing segments of the population to be infected with the virus, because women are more physiologically susceptible to HIV than men.

Further, the CDC tells us that African Americans account for 50 percent of new HIV cases each year, of which black women account for 72 percent. This number of infected black women may be connected to the secrecy of a huge bisexual segment of the population, who live basically "straight" lives, with exceptions. Their big dark secret is homosexual sex. They have a name for their sexual straying: they say they live life on the "down low." The Down Lows are teachers, rappers, preachers, lawyers, athletes, firemen, pilots, doctors, machinists, you name it. They come from a variety of racial and economic groups, but mostly they are African-American men.

A special stigma has always been attached to black men who have sex with men. Even now, when both society and legislation offer a measure of equality to both African Americans and homosexuals, black men suffer humiliation and alienation within their families, their churches, their business communities, their towns when they come out. And so they don't.

Men on the "down low" don't self-identify as gay or bisexual. But failing to admit to their behavior, even to themselves, means they don't plan for safe sex. So when the time comes, there they are with no condoms.

The community-mandated secrecy imposes a special kind of danger, because the female partners of the Down Lows are oblivious to their mates' "down low" behavior and often don't discover it until they themselves are infected. So terrified are these "up high" citizens that their carefully nurtured respectability will be blown, that they don't reveal their "down low" secrets to the women with whom they have sex—a fact that should cause wives and girlfriends to look more closely at the African-American men in their lives. (For more information, see the book *On the Down Low: A Journey Into the Lives of Straight Black Men Who Sleep With Men* and the film *No More Secrets, No More Lies*, both by J. L. King.)

Black or white, male or female, everyone needs to know that *AIDS is now the sixth leading cause of death among people between the ages of 15 and 24 in the United States.* You need to know how this deadly disease is spread, and you need to know how to protect yourself.

HIV is transmitted through sexual intercourse: homosexual (male-to-male and, though rarely, female-to-female) or heterosexual sex with a partner who is infected with HIV. It is also transmitted through needle-sharing. The exchange of bodily fluids from an infected partner to an uninfected partner is fundamental to transmission of the disease. Vaginal intercourse without a condom is the most common way the virus is transmitted between a man and a woman, although there are other ways. Oral sex can transmit the disease if the active partner has an open sore inside or outside his or her mouth. Anal intercourse without a condom can also transmit the disease. Danger of infection is more acute during anal than vaginal intercourse, but that's no excuse for having condom-less vaginal intercourse. It is still Russian roulette.

If you've had sex with *anybody*, it's possible you've contracted HIV. (As one of my currently celibate patients told me, "When I start dating again, the first date will be in the doctor's office with my new partner.") And if you've then had sex with someone who's not infected, it is possible you've passed the virus on. It's a pebble dropped into a pond. One ripple follows another and another and another.

How does it stop? You must help stop it.

If you have the slightest, the vaguest suspicion that you might be infected, get a test. Everyone should know their HIV status. The test can be done confidentially or anonymously. There are now rapid tests that give results in 20–30 minutes. If you are afraid of needles, there is a test that does not require blood to be taken. If you are very young and/or feel you have no one to turn to, call the CDC's National AIDS Hotline (800–342-AIDS) or go to a public health department.

There are Federally Qualified Community Health Centers (FQHC) in every state where you can get culturally and linguistically appropriate help, regardless of your immigration status or whether or not you have health insurance. Go to the next town if you fear for your anonymity in your own. Or go online for available testing information. It feels like you're alone, but you're not. There is confidential, professional, non-judgmental help available to you. And you must get help *because you must be tested*! (See the end of this book for more testing information).

Now, this is the hard part: you must inform your sexual partner or partners (present or past) what you've learned from your HIV test, if it is positive. If you don't tell, and you go on having unprotected sex, you're committing murder.

I know a man in his mid-forties who is HIV-positive. Since the onset of his illness he has been prescribed numerous medications, many of which he doesn't take regularly because the side effects are so debilitating. Consequently he has become highly resistant to many of the antiretrovirals. He is ill but determined to continue his active sex life with multiple partners, and without condoms. That determination is equaled only by his selfish negligence in telling his sexual partners he is HIV-positive. His physician knows this and is trying to get him to mend his homicidal behavior.

If you're simply unable to tell your partners because of embarrassment, most states provide free partner notification without identifying the infected person. The important thing is that you *don't wait* to get tested or to tell a partner that he or she needs to be tested. Don't wait for symptoms to show up. At first the virus can seem like a sniffly little cold, or the flu, maybe, with a rash, or fatigue, headache, perhaps a low-grade fever—the kind of ailment that certainly wouldn't make you think twice about making love or having sex. It's entirely possible you won't feel different at all, at first. There are no absolute, irrefutable, immediately recognizable symptoms of HIV, and a person can live with HIV symptoms for ten years before developing full-blown AIDS. Without an HIV test, that person won't know he or she is passing the virus on and on, and on. . . .

Make an appointment. Get the test. Make those calls. Use protection. That's how it stops.

CHAPTER FIVE

DO CONDOMS REALLY WORK?

47,000,000 infected, 0 cured

Without condom protection you are vulnerable to HIV transmission from vaginal, anal, or oral sex. According to the *Journal of Sexually Transmitted Diseases*, the risks of HIV transmission are 10,000 times greater among non-condom users than among the population that uses condoms all the time. Stated more optimistically, condom use during intercourse is 10,000 times safer than not using a condom.

The good news is this: used consistently and correctly, latex condoms are 98 percent effective. Therefore, to provide maximum protection, condoms must be used *consistently*, 100 percent of the time, and they must be used *correctly* 100 percent of the time. Unfortunately, 100 percent condom use is so unusual that the very idea of it is, for all intents and purposes, theoretical. However, one of my patients in her mid-thirties says she doesn't know what it feels like to have sex without a condom, since she never has. It can be done!—and must be done, because using condoms can save your life.

How do condoms prevent transmission of the AIDS virus? Simple: the virus that causes AIDS cannot penetrate latex. The virus is too large to escape latex pores. Condoms are double-dipped in latex, and the manufacturing process is so rigorous as to seem almost fanatical. The language on the packages—"triple tested," "individually electronically tested," "maximum reliability"—may sound like hype, but it's not. Different companies may use different methods to arrive at the efficacy of their products, and may advertise it using different terms. But whatever the language or methods, they all have identical standards to measure up to, standards set by that very tough taskmaster, the Food and Drug Administration (FDA). Those standards apply to all condoms sold in the United States, whether they are manufactured here or not.

Every condom approved by the FDA must pass an electric pinhole test, in which the condom is fitted onto a metal form called a mandrel in an intense electrical field. Rubber doesn't conduct electricity, so no electricity reaches the metal from under the condom unless the condom has a pinhole in it, in which case an indicator light goes off and the condom is rejected. The entire manufacturing lot in which that condom was found is tossed.

That's just one test.

There's a tensile test where equipment measures the condom's strength. The dimensions test precisely measures the length, width and thickness of a batch of condoms. When more than four out of 100 tested don't conform to an acceptable range, that entire lot from which the samples were taken is destroyed. There's an air burst properties test, a leakage test and a package integrity test, during which condom wrappers are checked for wrapper leaks.

Need more evidence that condoms are effective? Consider this: do you think Bill Gates would pour $200 million into a project that he didn't believe would work?

In December 2003, in Mysore, India, Bill and Melinda Gates began a program to provide information and condoms to those most at risk for contracting AIDS and passing it on—sex workers, soldiers, migrant workers, and truck drivers.* The information and condoms are

* In some states in India the prevalence of AIDS among prostitutes is 50 percent or greater. Truck drivers in India are ten times more likely than the general population to become infected with HIV (from having sex at truck stops). They then pass on the disease to their mates, who infect their unborn children.

distributed at clinics set up especially for the popula-tion at greatest risk. In sessions at these clinics, referred to as "Tea and Condoms," the audience is taught about safe sex, behavior modification, and HIV; and condoms are distributed. Health workers roam the streets to preach their condom/safe sex message, as well as to round up likely students for more comprehensive ses-sions at the clinics.

Just assembling citizenry to educate is not always easy, for India as a nation is shy about sex. The nation that produced the Kama Sutra, which emboldened many a generation to try stuff it never learned in sex education classes, doesn't want to discuss its famous export with health workers. Nonetheless, many anxious Indians are gratefully participating in long-overdue conversations about sex and reluctantly accepting gifts of condoms.* The project is still too new to have yield-ed statistics, but there's no shortage of evidence for the effectiveness of condoms.

For example, in 1986 in Uganda, the devastating AIDS epidemic started to slow when the country devel-oped a national campaign to accomplish a fundamental change in the nation's sexual behavior. The campaign

---

* Sex workers are fearful their husbands or families will discover condoms in their handbags, thus revealing their secret but desperately necessary careers. Poverty is its own disease.

was so simple, it seems almost impossible to believe that it worked. Referred to as the ABC, this is what it was: A. Abstain, and delay the age at which sexual activity commences. B. Be faithful. C. Use condoms if A and B fail. The president of Uganda often added D: if you don't do ABC you will die. The success of the program in Uganda (a decrease in new HIV cases from 20 percent a year to 6 percent from 1992 to 2000) can be largely attributed to the country's president, who believed in it and put resources behind it. The next chapter, "The Politics of Condoms," describes another successful approach in Brazil.

A 1993 U.S. study published in the *Journal of Acquired Immune Deficiency Syndromes* found that among 171 uninfected women having sex with HIV-infected partners (called discordant couples) who used condoms, only two contracted the virus. That's about 1.2 percent. In another study about the same time, eight out of ten women whose partners didn't use condoms every time became infected. That's *80 percent.*

It's no secret that *condoms are the best protection against the transmission of the Human Immunodeficiency Virus that technology currently offers.* Yet only 87 percent of discordant couples do not use condoms consistently. Is it any wonder people are dying by the millions?

Individuals must act responsibly to stop this disease. However, responsible action requires information and access to options. In some places—maybe closer than you think—information and options are being blocked, and people are dying. What you are about to read will make you angry, but it could also save your life.

CHAPTER SIX

THE POLITICS OF CONDOMS

47,000,000 infected, 0 cured

The nature of sex is anarchic—unpredictable, reckless, hard to control—and so it has long been an issue for the institutions that try to bring order to the citizenry. Religions, governments, and schools have created rules, laws, punishments, and restrictions in order to control sexual behavior and make the lawmakers feel empowered.

Condoms as a method of sexual disease prevention are a medical fact; however, when they are issued or withheld by government bodies, they often become a political football in the courts of public opinion. The actions of government vis-à-vis sex are usually not only idiotic but dangerous. Prisons are perfect examples of places where sexual rules run amok.

Only a few jail systems in the United States distribute condoms. The Los Angeles County Jail began distributing to declared gay inmates in September 2002, joining four other municipal jail systems and two state systems: New York City, Philadelphia, Washington, San Francisco, Vermont, and Mississippi. Other correctional facilities in the United States don't distribute condoms, and they have three reasons for not doing so: condoms could be used as weapons; condoms could be used to hide smuggled goods; and their distribution seems to suggest that homosexual sex is okay, even permitted.

Canada has made condoms available to prisoners since 1992. When questioned about the first two reasons for not distributing them in American prisons, Ralf Jurgens, director of the Canadian HIV/AIDS Legal Network, indicated that no such problems had ever arisen in Canadian correctional facilities. The third reason—that in distributing condoms, American prisons seem to be condoning homosexual sex—is a denial of reality, the lethal effects of which extend far beyond any prison system that fears the appearance of being soft on homosexual sex.

Prisons are incubators and disseminators of HIV. The U.S. prison population totaled 2,078,570 at the end of 2003. While the majority of men entering prison would self-identify as heterosexual, many leave with a history of multiple same-sex experiences, which has led in many cases to HIV. When HIV-positive prisoners are released, they share the disease with wives and girlfriends as well as other members of the general population. This is neither a secret nor news.

Given this frightening reality, you would think state and federal prisons might distribute condoms. But prison authorities continue to refuse to acknowledge that sex occurs in prisons. As a result, year after year the prison system continues to function as a major contributor to AIDS in the general population, as people leaving prison carry HIV to the unsuspecting outside world.

A grandmother of four came to ask my advice on how to tell her granddaughters that their mother was dying of AIDS. "She is my only daughter, an only child, as I was, and she never knew her father," this lady told me. "She always said, 'When I have children they are going to know their father.' She was determined. We all think that's why she stayed with him, although he was in and out of prison." She was angry that this man had given her only child AIDS, and depressed that her daughter had kept it a secret until it was too late.

I kept thinking, *We can do better than this.*

Abstinence is the official right-wing solution to all sexual problems. The further the politician is to the right, the greater his or her faith in chastity. Now, as I've said, abstinence/chastity is high on my list of answers to the war against HIV/AIDS. Yet, in 25 years of medical practice, I have not run into it too often. As a solution to a deadly worldwide plague, abstinence advocacy is the medical version of whistling in the dark.

In a culture bombarded by sexuality in film, television, print, even radio, there is still tremendous resistance to providing sex education, information, or advice, let alone condoms to those on the brink of their sexual lives. Any realistic view of young people would suggest that school children should start learning about condom use at the age of ten, since sexual activity often begins at age twelve. A study from the BBC News, presented at the 2004 National STD Conference in Philadelphia, examined the sex lives of 12,000 adolescents aged 12–18. According to the study, the STD rates were the same for those who pledged virginity as for those who didn't. The author's message is simple: in the long term, "Just say no" doesn't work.

An interesting measure of comparative conservatism of the two Bush administrations was given by

Nicholas Kristof in his January 10, 2003 column in the *New York Times*. He pointed out that the number of condoms the United States contributes worldwide dropped from 800 million at the end of the first President Bush's term to 300 million currently.

As an alarming matter of fact, the CDC has been publishing misleading statistics on the effectiveness of condoms. Since the CDC is a branch of the federal government, it is also under the federal government's jurisdiction, and the current president strongly believes in "harm avoidance," i.e., no sex at all, rather than "harm reduction." So cooking the statistics may be bad science but good politics. As the *New York Times* has said, "In this administration, politics trumps science!" To its credit, when the CDC's inaccurate statistics were challenged it corrected them to correspond to the reality of the efficacy of condoms.

Even television networks, which show people copulating like crazy on screen, undressing, murdering, torturing, violating each other in unspeakable ways, have maintained strict standards about permitting condom advertising. ABC, UPN, and the WB TV network won't permit condom advertising at all. Fox, CBS, and NBC do show condom commercials, originally only on late, late shows, but now thankfully in prime time—a golden viewing time that has long welcomed commercials for racy underwear and Viagra.

There is actually one commercial about condoms especially worth noting—it played on the radio, in Texas—and that commercial is a lie: "Condoms will not protect people from many sexually transmitted diseases." Similarly, in October 2003, a high Vatican official told the BBC's *Panorama* program that the latex condom contains pores that will not stop the transmission of HIV. Ironically, no organization on earth does more for AIDS victims than the Catholic church. Yet it continues to promote this narrow thinking.

Information about this disease is so precious that a church, a college, a political party that withholds information about sex, HIV/AIDS, condoms, or sexual behavior—or, in some cases, withholds condoms—is essentially condemning people to death. The number of people such "official-speak" condemns to death depends on the size and power of the controlling group. It could be a few, it could be hundreds, or it could be tens of millions.

Public policy about HIV/AIDS should be untainted by politics and geared to the population that honestly wants to protect itself. Sadly, this may not be everybody. The message to use condoms would be much more forceful and focused if it ignored the hard-core nihilists who don't want help and who are indifferent about transmitting the virus. Adopting the mantra "Look beautiful, live fast, die young," some individuals squander themselves at so-called "poz parties," "conversion parties," and "gift-giving parties," where they go to have sex with anybody who wants to play. Often they are already infected with HIV/AIDS and feel they have nothing to lose by having unprotected sex (called "barebacking"), or they are uninfected but tired of the effort to prevent becoming infected. Two consenting adults should be free to share their virus, but only if there are NO public consequences to their private actions.

This part of the population needs special help. But they are often no more receptive to the message that they need help than drug addicts are to the message "Just say no." And sometimes, to avoid excluding them, we couch AIDS prevention messages in terms that are wispy-murky or cute and coy, instead of clear and pragmatic. There is a socio-medical term, "herd immunity," that applies to the percentage of the population that medicine thinks it can save with immunization. With the immunization of that percentage, the other, much smaller percentage won't be able to transmit the disease to those behaving responsibly. That same thinking, applied to condom education and condom use, would go a long way to helping stem the HIV/AIDS pandemic. This is a far greater challenge than immunization.

Clearly, official public policy inspired by true public spirit is a good beginning. The CDC should be commended for one key part of its new strategy: to reduce new HIV infections by urging every person to know his or her status. Many of my patients, however, have the misconception that the test carries with it some kind of protection. Of course it does not. What it does do is help a person make an informed choice: to get treatment, if infected, and to use condoms, whether infected or not.

In the arena of public good, money, of course, is always an issue. Using on average one condom a day, a year's supply of condoms would cost about $365.00. Compare that to the $12,000 to $15,000 annual cost of treating one HIV-infected person—which doesn't include the other medical and social costs that go beyond the cost of medication. Some health insurance companies actually have the wisdom to pay for condoms.

An easy and inexpensive expression of public spirit would be distribution of condoms in appropriate places: bath houses, sex clubs, and in all the places where sanitary products are dispensed. In New York, legislation has been introduced to require condoms in every hotel room. They may remain as untouched as the Gideon Bible, but they may not. Think of the good they could do.

Currently, according to a May 18, 2004 *New York Times* editorial, our federal government is simultaneously helping those infected with AIDS and thwarting help for those at high risk for becoming infected. For example, the government is expediting a review by the FDA of a new pill that purports to help individuals infected with AIDS. The pill, cheaper and simpler to take than previously available medication, could save lives that would otherwise be lost to AIDS. On the other hand, AIDS prevention—my mission—is being politicized and dangerously shunted aside by the Bush administration. In a deep bow to the powerful religious right, one third of this country's AIDS-prevention funds has been allotted to abstinence-only programs, in spite of the fact that such programs by themselves aren't successful. Justification for this puzzler comes from Randall Tobias, the administration's AIDS coordinator, who insists condoms are ineffective. He uses as his authority the London School of Hygiene and Tropical Medicine, which not only denies having produced the report he quotes but in fact says that condoms do indeed work to prevent AIDS.

The websites for the CDC and the Agency for International Development no longer contain information about condom use or the value of sex education, thanks to the removal of such education by our current administration.

All nations aren't so narrow and shortsighted, however. For Carnival in Rio, in 2003, Brazil's Ministry of Health distributed 20 million "little shirts" (condoms) to assure a healthier celebration. The World Bank predicted in 1992 that 1.2 million people in Brazil would be living with HIV by 2002. (Brazil's population is 170 million.) The public health measures adopted by Brazil were so effective that the number today is just 215,000—17 percent of the World Bank's grim projection.

Success is possible, even in a large country with a large, complex population, when the government neither judges, winces, nor wimps out when administering help to stop the world's most devastating pandemic.

CHAPTER SEVEN

CONDOMS: PLANNING, PROTEC-
TION AND PEACE OF MIND

47,000,000 infected, 0 cured

Wen I set out to write this book, it was all about the prevention of HIV through the use of condoms. Then I met a young woman who changed my mind. The message about condom use to prevent other sexually transmitted diseases and unwanted pregnancies needs to be restated.

The young woman to whom I refer came in to be treated for some minor ailment. With this patient, as with all others, I took advantage of the opportunity to do an assessment of the risk behaviors in which she may have generally engaged. So I asked the usual questions about sexual activity, sexual preference, and use of contraceptives. At first, this 18-year-old said that she practiced abstinence. I then asked if she was a virgin. She explained that she had had three abortions, and had decided not to have sex anymore. I encouraged her born-again virginity. I next asked her what form of birth control she would consider in place of abortion in the event that she changed her mind about abstinence. She burst into tears and cried uncontrollably for five minutes. I apologized and said that I had not meant to make her cry. Her response was, "It's not you."

Somewhere along the way the message has been communicated to this young woman that she must avoid having a child at all cost, yet somehow she never learned how to protect herself from the risks of sex—STDs, HIV, sterility, emotional stress, even death. Was she in one of the thousands of school districts that won't permit sex education or condom distribution (both of which are very common prohibitions, and not just in the Bible belt)? Had she ever been taught the relationship between alcohol use and sexual activity? Did anyone ever teach her refusal skills? Did anyone show her love?

As a society, we have failed this young woman, and it weighs heavily on me.

The numbers are staggering. Seventy-five percent of the babies born to adolescents are unplanned and untimely. Thirty-three percent of pregnancies among 15- to 19-year-olds in the United States are terminated by abortion. How much simpler it would be to prevent pregnancy in the frist place than to have to make that painful decision after one is pregnant! As the former Surgeon General Dr. Jocelyn Elders said, "I've never heard of anyone needing an abortion who wasn't pregnant." She further commented that just as we teach kids how to behave in the front of the car, we should teach them how to behave in the back seat.

It has been well documented in study after study that teaching adolescents how to use condoms correctly does not encourage them to have sex any more than carrying an umbrella causes rain. In many places in the United States adolescents can obtain contraceptive advice without the consent of their parents. The problem is that many adolescents lack insurance coverage independent of their parents and therefore cannot get the help they need. (See the information on Community Health Centers in the resource section at the back of this book.)

The advantages of the male latex condom for contraception are numerous and comforting.

- Condoms are ready when you are.
- Condoms do double duty—contraception as well as protection against HIV, gonorrhea, syphilis, trichomoniasis, chlamydia, and many other diseases. Condoms are most effective against the diseases associated with a discharge.
- Condoms are safe even if you smoke, unlike birth control pills.
- Condoms do not cause weight gain, unlike birth control pills or hormone injections.
- Condoms do not have to be put on or in ahead of time.
- Condom use can be easily incorporated into sexual foreplay.
- Condoms have no side effects if you are not allergic to latex. (For more information on what to do if you or your partner has a latex allergy, see Chapter 8.)
- Condoms are inexpensive.
- Condoms are stored easily.
- Condoms pack and carry easily.
- Condoms are readily available. No prescription is needed.
- Condoms provide disease protection for vaginal, oral and anal sex.
- Condoms provide birth control that can be ended

simply by stopping their use. With hormonal contraceptive methods (like birth control pills, or Depo Provera injections) you have to stop taking them months before a planned pregnancy in order to give eggs time to develop.

- Condoms aren't messy like spermicidal creams and jellies, and are more effective.
- Condoms don't make your periods heavy like an intrauterine device (IUD).
- Condoms can be used at any age, by adolescents, geriatrics, and everyone in between.
- Condoms are 98 percent effective when used properly from start to finish every time you have sex.

Condoms can break. If you are concerned about becoming pregnant, the contraceptive morning-after pill is still available and is most effective if taken within 72 hours. At the time of this writing, there is a move afoot to make the contraceptive morning-after pill available over the counter, without a prescription. There is a pilot project in Seattle, Washington, that sells oral contraception to women without a prescription after a health survey is completed and their blood pressure taken. (For treatment to prevent HIV infection in the event that a condom breaks, see Chapter 8.)

When thinking of the utility of condoms, I am reminded of an interview with the 2,000-Year-Old Man (Mel Brooks). The character is asked what he considers to be the most important medical breakthrough over his lifetime. The 2,000-Year-Old Man thinks for a while and then answers, "Liquid Prell." The interviewer is astonished. "In light of such breakthroughs as the Salk Vaccine, penicillin, and the heart-lung machine, how can you elevate Liquid Prell to such an honored position?" he asks. "Do you really think Liquid Prell deserves this honor?" "Yes, yes I do," answers the 2,000-Year-Old Man. "If you put the heart-lung machine in a medicine cabinet, it could fall on you and kill you. Liquid Prell won't even break."

My candidate for the greatest technological invention of the past 2,000 years is the condom. It's what the world needs now and it's what my patient needed and so many others like her.

CHAPTER EIGHT

CONDOMS: HOW TO CHOOSE THEM, HOW TO USE THEM

47,000,000 infected, 0 cured

U sed consistently and correctly, condoms are life-savers. Their effectiveness therefore depends on the individual. Embarrassment is no longer an excuse, nor is uncertainty, ignorance, drunkenness, drugs, inexperience, or clumsiness.

When purchasing condoms, pay attention to the packaging. Check the expiration date. Has the condom been stored at the correct temperature (is the display counter in the sun, by a heater or under a harsh light)? Too much heat will weaken condoms and render them useless. Is the package itself securely closed?

Store your own condoms at room temperature (72

degrees), and not in your wallet. Carry them in your wallet, of course; they're a time-honored symbol of hope. But don't make it a permanent storage place. And don't put them where a practical joker can get to them for his own sadistic fun.

The first time you put on a condom shouldn't be the first time you use a condom. Whatever manner of sex you're using it for, you must know how to put one on correctly and safely. Anal sex poses a special risk of condom failure the first few times it occurs, unless the condom-wearing partner puts the condom on the right way, which means the safe way. So, in private, with no nervous expectations, no one waiting in the next room or on the other side of the bed, you must practice the condom routine. If it seems like a lot of trouble, well, it's for your own good, and for your partner's good. What better way to show your concern? It's a matter of life or death. Besides, learning to put on a condom will lessen the nervousness of the moment. Looking like you know what you're doing will help you avoid embarrassment—or failure to achieve success when you really, really want success.

But what about spontaneity, exuberance, that just-for-the-hell-of-it, devil-may-care rainy afternoon, the all-of-a-sudden, unexpected, fabulous, unplanned-for moment, in the back of a car, on the office floor, under the piano, in a sun-drenched meadow, a memory you'll carry with you for the rest of your life? Prepare for that moment by practicing *now*. Wearing a condom doesn't mean sex can't be spontaneous, exciting, romantic— since condom wear is so important, why not incorporate it into your sex life as part of foreplay? If you involve your mate in the process, the process itself becomes more interesting, and more mutually responsible.

But *before* you involve your mate in the process, you need to know what you're doing, starting with the opening of a condom package. Even before you put on a condom you must exercise care. Putting on a condom safely and successfully begins with opening the package correctly, so there's no damage to the condom. Impatience can mean death. Fingernails or teeth will create rips, making the condom useless, maybe even murderous. Just ease it gently into a corner of its package, then open the package and carefully remove the condom.

To put a condom on you must have an erection. Be certain to pinch the closed end of the condom to eliminate any air trapped inside, and to leave room for the ejaculation ("cum"). An uncircumcised man must pull back his foreskin before putting on a condom. Then, start slipping it on, sort of like a sock, unrolling it very,

very carefully. Then smooth out any bubbles that may still be in the condom. The instructions are on all the condom packages, clearly, succinctly written. But who reads them?

Rehearse this over and over, not to look like a smooth operator, though there's nothing wrong with that, but to do it absolutely right every single time you put it on. And of course *you will put a condom on every single time you have penetrative sex, every single time, no excuses, start to finish.*

Using a household lubricant—like Vaseline, mineral oil, vegetable oil, cold cream or hand lotion—can be a deadly mistake. Research shows that within 60 seconds petroleum-based lubricants can erode a condom so much that it's useless. Use a water-based lubricant, such as K-Y jelly, to make sex more comfortable and help prevent condoms from ripping.

Some condoms come already lubricated with a water-based spermicide, which provides a little more ease and comfort than unlubricated condoms, but no significant additional safeguard against HIV transmission. Until recently, pharmaceutical spermicides such as Nonoxonyl-9 were recommended as an added protection against HIV/AIDS. New research shows, however, that spermicides offer no protection against these viruses. They can even cause harm if they irritate the vagina or the rectum, thus making the transmission of the virus easier. (Nonoxynol-9 has earned the particular disapproval of the WHO and the CDC in this regard; other spermicides are also questionable but have not been examined as closely or critically.) However, if it's Saturday night and the stores are closed and you have neither latex nor polyurethane condoms, but you do have a spermicide, use the spermicide. It's better than nothing, unless the spermicide is Nonoxynol-9. One third of condoms produced in the United States are lubricated with spermicides, most often with Nonoxynol-9. Because of the potential for irritation and virus transmission, or even allergic reaction, avoid these condoms.

Removing a condom is a little harder to practice, so pay attention to make certain that you do it the right way. When you're finished, take the condom off before your penis softens, being careful not to spill the contents. Then empty the condom into the toilet, and, so nobody tries to reuse it, tie a knot in it before tossing it into the trash.

Make sure you use a fresh condom every time you engage in penetrative sex, whether the sex is oral, anal, or vaginal. Many gay men use condoms for anal but not oral sex. Big mistake. Anal sex, oral sex—condom, every single time, start to finish.

There's a syndrome around called "condom fatigue." It was first named and noted in Canadian research and has since picked up steam in America. Condom fatigue was first misguidedly linked to homosexual sex. It actually pertains best to teen-age and college-age populations. The term describes the explosion of condom use during first-time sexual experiences, which later diminishes as young people grow more experienced, or more jaded, about their sexual experiences.

The best way to avoid becoming jaded about sex is to be abstinent. Not only is abstinence the best way to avoid AIDS, it's a wonderful way to keep the act of sex and the idea of sex fresh, vivid, and ecstatic until you are ready for a committed relationship. Of course, if abstinence were more popular I'd be the happiest doctor in America and wouldn't be writing this book. But, as I've witnessed too terribly and too often, it's a lovely dream. Unplanned pregnancies, 600,000 thrown away children (children in foster care) in the United States and a world population of almost 6 billion people, with approximately 47 million of them infected with HIV, demonstrate that clearly enough.

What to Do About a Latex Allergy

Up to 17 percent of health care workers whose careers are inseparable from latex gloves are allergic to latex, but only about one percent of the general population is allergic to latex. Allergic reactions to latex gloves are generally more severe than to latex condoms. The symptoms (in varying degrees of intensity) include itching, eczema, skin rash, and dryness.

Before you place the blame for your discomfort on a latex condom, consider your recent sex life. If you've had more than your normal amount of intercourse, perhaps it's not latex but irritation due to the friction of the additional activity.

Take a sex break for a couple of days and wash with cool water (don't use soap). If whatever is bothering you doesn't clear up, consult a health-care professional. Or try this if you suspect a latex condom is the culprit: pull on a latex glove. If your hand reacts with a mild tingling or itching, you have a latex problem. The discomfort from latex is called contact dermatitis. A gynecologist I spoke with assured me that latex condom allergies are rare and usually mild.

If you have not seen a medical professional but are about to resume your sex life, make certain you use a lubricant (not a petroleum-based lubricant) along with the latex condom. If the itching continues or resumes, you probably have a latex allergy.

Latex allergies can be handled by doing something called "double sheathing." First, put on a lambskin condom, then over it a latex condom—or vice versa, depending on which partner is latex-sensitive. An ultra-sheer latex condom will help compensate for the cumbersome layering effect of two condoms. That way you'll be protected from HIV (which the lambskin condom can't do alone) and from the latex allergy, without sacrificing pleasure.

Some medical professionals recommend the female polyurethane condom when one partner has a latex allergy. For more information, see Chapter 11.

If Your Condom Breaks During Intercourse

It happens infrequently, but it does happen. Studies in the United States indicate that the breakage rate is 2 condoms out of every 100. A condom may break if it's old or has been stored incorrectly, if you've used the wrong kind of lubricant, if the condom is too small, or if the sex act itself is unusually active or athletic. All those reasons notwithstanding, the primary reason for breakage is putting the condom on incorrectly.

If the condom breaks, stay calm. Do an assessment of the situation. Don't douche the vagina or anus. Don't even give yourself a little sponge bath. You may, however, urinate if the break occurs during vaginal sex. What you must not do is shrug it off and take a "well, next time I'll make certain it doesn't break" approach. If you're having sex with someone who you know is HIV-positive, or whose sexual health you're in the dark about, and your condom (or his condom) breaks, get yourself immediately to an HIV expert (see the Resource section at the end of this book), who will probably put you on medication for six weeks. (This is based on the post-exposure prophylaxis for occupational exposure.) At the end of six weeks, if you're not positive, you will be taken off the medication.

If your partner's antibody test is still negative (apparently not infected with HIV, or possibly infected but the virus has not yet emerged), go on medication at least as long as his status is unknown. Again, postexposure prophylaxis must be carried out under the care of an HIV expert. The practice that is most pervasive on the street is to take an antiretroviral pill, pro vided by a friend or bought on the black market, after participating in unsafe sex. This is not a solution.

This is serious stuff. Casual is no longer a word that can be applied to sexual activity, however casual your feelings. Behave responsibly. The health of the world is at stake, and you have a role in it.

CHAPTER NINE

CHANGING CONDOM ATTITUDES

47,000,000 infected, 0 cured

When mass-produced condoms first came on the scene in 1844, during the Victorian Age, abstinence and coitus interruptus ("withdrawal") were the norm. Not surprisingly, these methods met with stunning failure. Sexually transmitted diseases flourished, and many unwanted children were born. Though the Victorians were among the world's most sexually obsessed people, any public mention of sex was met with horror and condemnation. So, sneaking around became synonymous with a sex life.

In those days, there was no swaggering or sneaking into a pharmacy to ask for condoms. They were discreetly procured from a forward-thinking doctor or pharmacist, and were used ostensibly for the prevention of diseases acquired from prostitutes. Wives, who would have adored something that would prevent pregnancy and disease while keeping their husbands happy in bed at home, were simply not condom privy.

The secrecy and embarrassment continued through the 1950s. A young man out to buy a condom would ditch his plans for the evening rather than buy condoms from a female pharmacy clerk. Or he'd sit at the soda fountain killing time until she took a cigarette break and a man took over at the counter. This bashful behavior continued for decades because of disapproval over sex and anything that had anything to do with sex.

Ask your grandparents when they first heard the word "condom," or were even aware that there was such a thing. They knew nothing at an age when you think you know everything. But what in those times people liked to think of as "innocence" was more akin to blind ignorance. (What would be true innocence in a child is ignorance at an age when you should know better.) Americans and sexual ignorance are old, old friends, and the friendship continues today in this world of apparent sexual liberation and openness.

During the First World War the secretary of the navy forbade the distribution of condoms to sailors on the grounds that to use condoms was immoral and "unChristian." (Think of all those young, testosterone-driven sailors released onto foreign ports with nothing but memories of Sunday school lessons to protect them.) The wise young assistant secretary of the navy, Franklin Delano Roosevelt, countermanded his boss's orders, and American sailors went into foreign ports with condoms and dreams.

As late as the Second World War, however, American soldiers were still flinging themselves over the sides of troop carriers armed with nothing but their weapons. (The English military were given condoms as well as their regular allotment of whisky before entering foreign countries.) As the war wore on, America's military leaders woke up and supplied servicemen with condoms after showing them a film with the slogan, "Put it on before you put it in." (Many of those condoms were used to protect rifle barrels from getting wet during landings.)

Perhaps surprisingly, the Sexual Revolution of the '60s and '70s, which changed life in both straight and gay communities—when "good girls" did the things only "bad girls" had previously had the nerve to do—actually brought to a screeching halt the sale of condoms. Who needed them? Condoms were for fuddy-duddies. Let the unprotected sex begin!

With the appearance of HIV and AIDS, in the '80s and '90s, attitudes about protection were turned around yet again, full circle.

A physician in Brooklyn kept a cookie jar in her home for her young family. When the kids grew into teenagers the cookies in the jar were replaced by condoms, available to anybody with the good sense to want them.

The same doctor gave a lecture to some senior citizens about using protection for safe sex. One oldster, proud as proud, stood up and announced that condoms were just too damn restrictive for a guy as gorgeously endowed—as, let's face it, big—as he. As he spoke the doctor was fiddling behind the podium with her right arm. At the close of this little speech, the doctor held up her right arm sheathed from fist to elbow in a condom. "Bigger than this?" she asked.

For young men and women alike, the age of blushing when buying condoms is as old-fashioned as celibacy. There is, however, an occasional odd exception. I once knew a well-educated man in his fifties who fell in love with a woman, also in her fifties. When asked by his doctor what kind of protection he used, he almost blushed, and replied, "I don't use any." Apparently he had gone into a pharmacy for the express purpose of buying condoms, but when he saw a crowd of sedate women near the condom section—they were taking their blood pressure at the nearby blood pressure machine—he fled, and never returned to that pharmacy again. Eventually his doctor gave him a lecture and a supply of condoms for the weekend, instructing him to buy online.

He isn't a typical modern man. The folks in the following tale, however, are typical.

A young couple in a small neighborhood grocery store stood at the head of a long and getting-longer line arguing about the merits of the condoms they were buying.

"No, I hate this one," said she.

"You used to like it," said he. "What happened?"

"Nothing. That's what happened."

And so it went while the line got longer and longer, stretching from the checkout counter way back to the frozen beans.

CHAPTER TEN

THE NEW SEXUAL DIPLOMACY: NEGOTIATING CONDOM WEAR

47,000,000 infected, 0 cured

"**W**hat'll I do if he tries to kiss me?" On that first date, this used to be the big question—if not for our mothers, certainly for our grandmothers. Many a young girl felt compromised because she let down the bar and not only permitted a kiss, but kissed back—and, worse, liked it. As social mores changed regarding sex, the question became, "Should I go to bed with him on the first date?" And then, with the advent of AIDS, "How do I get him to use a condom when we go to bed?"

There are lots of cute answers to the condom question that don't deserve attention because it's not a cute question. Likewise, humility and uncertainty have no place in the new sexual environment. It's a question of life or death.

You would think, wouldn't you, unless you were married, and were hoping to have children, that wearing a condom would be as natural as brushing your teeth. It shouldn't require diplomacy or negotiation. It should be a shared responsibility, in which you keep a supply of condoms on hand and your mate either has his own or doesn't resist when you show him your supply. That's how it should be.

Often it's the man who takes the offensive. "What have you been doing that you want me to wear a condom?" Women who know that their mate is unfaithful often say, "I hope when he's out there he's doing the right thing." Translated, this means, "I hope he's wearing a condom."

Like many, many situations between men and women, the condom-ready situation has changed. You no longer have to hope your guy will cooperate and wear a condom. You no longer have to fret over the condom debate. There doesn't have to be a debate.

Even if you are married, you have a right to request that your husband wear a condom.

If the request angers him and he forces himself on

you, that's rape. "Rape is not a shame, it's a crime." By law, a woman does not have to submit to her husband's violent whims. Today, society esteems women's courage and the value women place on their bodies. Husband or not, wives are under no obligation to leave the decision to wear a condom up to the man. In my practice, women sometimes say, "I just give in to keep the family together." Who is going to keep the family together if you die of AIDS? Most women of childbearing age who die of AIDS leave three dependent children.

You must not feel for a scintilla of a second that you are asking a man to compromise his fun. (Some people claim sex with a condom "just doesn't feel as good." Would dying feel better?) You must not fumble, mumble, stumble around, hoping to arrive at an amenable joint condom attitude. And you certainly shouldn't wait until the last minute, when you're in the bedroom, because by then nobody's thinking straight.

This firm stance is not, of course, limited to men and women, husbands and wives. Sex workers, too, must successfully negotiate condom wear. The world's oldest profession certainly deserves protection and dignity under the law, which it has in many nations, including Denmark, Australia, the Philippines, Canada, France,

Israel, and others. But in the United States, except for some counties in Nevada, prostitution is still illegal. Precisely because of its unlawful status, those of you who ply this ancient profession have an obligation to protect yourselves. In doing so, you also protect your clients and the mates you truly love. Not only must you supply condoms for your clients if they don't have them, but you must resist when clients have bad ideas— "I don't wear condoms," for example. In that case, the deal is off. No condoms, no deal, no fun. That's what you and all your peers must do.

Now, here's an idea that goes further, will actually make your life easier, and may even promote a sisterhood between you and your fellow sex workers. Why not mobilize and agree that you won't serve your clients without condoms? That way the guys can't turn to another girl and give her HIV/AIDS, or get it from her. Pimps, too, if they balk at condom use, should be reminded that with compliance they won't get sick from sex with their employees, nor will their employees get sick from them. Your new sisterhood will be your own government, exercising some control over your own lives. Of course, the federal government should perform this function, but until it does (don't hold your breath), try making your own health-generating rules.

Homosexuals engaging in sex with strangers, even sex with a loved one, must also take a firm, no-debate stand on condom use—not to question or insult your companion, but to protect you both. The right and necessity of condom wear is obvious, and you can make a case for it very clearly. If the message doesn't seem to get through, or if it meets with obdurate resistance, then pass the opportunity by and say good-bye.

Clear-headedness is key to the new sexual diplomacy. Do not be misled by drugs, alcohol, or moonlight. You must not be a victim of your state of mind. Safe, healthy sexual behavior should happen with forethought, foresight, and planning. Keep a ready supply of your own condoms—at home, in your handbag or briefcase, in your desk, in your backpack. With caution like this, you won't suffer morning-after regrets or terrors. Your condoms should be as accessible as lipstick or a cell phone. (A billboard in New York City says, "92 percent of you carry lip protection, 10 percent of you carry protection against HIV.") And considering how condoms have changed from those plain old "rubbers" of history to condoms with definite embellishments— textures, colors, fragrances, tastes, built-in excitement (literally)—you could even make the condom selection a part of foreplay.

An older, church-going woman, in answer to my question about her sexual activity, shrugged. Her shrug indicated she had no love life. The shrug changed to a nervous wiggle in her chair and downcast eyes. No love life except . . . the father of her child had recently waltzed into her life after 25 years—25 years of who knows what funny business. Then one thing led to another—he is, after all, the father of her child, which to her granted him automatic bedding privileges—and she couldn't summon the nerve to ask him to wear a condom. So of course he didn't and of course she went to bed with him.

Guess what? He's gone again. She has accepted HIV counseling and testing.

Instead of surrendering to the father of her child, she would have made her life easier if she had responded the way one of my other patients did when confronted with a reluctant condom-wearer.

He said to her, "I can't feel it if I wear a condom."

She said to him, *"You're not going to feel it if you don't."*

She has never had to be tested for HIV.

CHAPTER ELEVEN

THE FEMALE CONDOM: EQUALITY BETWEEN THE SHEETS?

47,000,000 infected, 0 cured

Fifteen thousand years after the first sighting of a male condom (in Upper Paleolithic cave paintings in Combarelles, France), women finally have a condom of their very own—designed for the female anatomy, female peace of mind, and female empowerment. At last women won't have to surrender their sexuality to male prejudices or whims, won't have to depend on technology honed for guys by guys.

Introducing the condom made just for women.

Ta-daa! Or ... ta-daa?

The new condom for women should be a breakthrough. But this new addition to female sexual independence has undergone some scrutiny—and inspired some head scratching.

First, the basics: the female condom is made of polyurethane, a strong material so soft and so thin that it conducts heat, which makes intercourse feel more natural and allows increased sensitivity—and, of course, more excitement. The Reality Condom and the FC Female Condom are the brands that have been market-ed in this country; the FC Female Condom replaced the name Reality a couple of years ago. In Europe the same design is called Femidon, but in other parts of the world it is still called Reality. Femidon, FC and Reality are all manufactured in the United States by the Female Health Company.

Now, why the scrutiny? Why the head scratching?

In 1991 the FDA approved polyurethane for male condoms as well as for the new female condom. Then, in 1993, that status was revoked, polyurethane having failed to live up to the FDA's rigorous standards. Female condoms would still be marketed, but with restrictive labeling stating that women's polyurethane condoms offer *limited* protection against STDs, and that for highly effective protection against STDs, including AIDS, it is important to use latex condoms for men.

Since 1993, there have been no announcements indicating an FDA change of status for polyurethane. As a result, medical journals, women's health newsletters, and university publications have all held back their approval of the female condom's efficacy. Indeed, this should make any woman think seriously about its use as a defense against the virus that causes AIDS. However, as birth control, and for protection against sexually transmitted diseases, the female condom continues to have its proponents.

As of this writing (2004), many doctors continue to recommend the female condom for patients with latex allergies, and because FDA approval appears imminent. But until an official announcement is made, it is important to realize that even the label on the female condom itself suggests using latex condoms instead of polyurethane if you're not allergic to latex: "Latex condoms for men are highly effective at preventing sexually transmitted diseases, including AIDS (HIV infection), if used properly. If you are not going to use a male latex condom, you can use the female condom to help protect yourself and your partner." Online sources for answers to questions about safe sex take their cue from this carefully worded statement and say, "The female condom is certainly an option and provides more protection than using nothing at all," or "If the fact that polyurethane condoms do not yet have full FDA approval concerns you, try using ultra-thin latex condoms, which may be more heat conductive than regular latex, until full FDA approval is granted to polyurethane condoms."

Still, because the polyurethane of the female condom protects against allergic reactions, many medical advisors and journals regard it as a viable alternative to latex, the "next best thing." As you might guess, that gives me pause.

There are other problems, too. The National Library of Medicine reports a study relating to rates of slippage and breakage of polyurethane and latex condoms. Polyurethane lost on both counts. The polyurethane condom's clinical breakage rate was 7.2 percent to the latex condom's 1.1 percent. However, for sheer pleasure of the moment, the subjects in the study preferred polyurethane because of its heat-conducting thinness. Note: ultra-thin latex also provides heat-conducting thinness. (If "ultra-thin" connotes fragility to you, put the thought from your head. Ultra-thinness compromises neither strength nor safety.)

Also, the female condom is quite funny looking—daunting, even, compared to the mindless simplicity of the male condom's design. It's a very thin and floppy sheath, lubricated inside and out, with a ring at either end. The ring that fits into the vagina is enclosed and is inserted like a diaphragm. The way the FC fits, of course, is crucial; sometimes the fit is loose enough that the penis penetrates outside it, providing zero protection.

Still, the female condom isn't without its advantages. Any kind of lubricant can be applied, water- or oil-based, without compromising the integrity of the device. It can be inserted some time before having sex, unlike the male condom, and that's an excellent thing, because it forestalls the last-minute angst that inserting the condom could entail. Pre-intercourse insertion also effectively eliminates the negotiations that can accompany male condoms (see Chapter 10). And that is perhaps the reason for its popularity among disenfranchised female populations. (It is currently available in 30 countries.) In Africa, for example, approval of the female condom is unguarded and enthusiastic; its efficacy is lauded for birth control and for protection against STDs and HIV. The idea of a female condom is certainly empowering, especially for women who, in most or parts of their lives, feel overwhelmingly unempowered. Women can protect themselves, according to the FDA, "without depending on the cooperation of their partners." Never mind that the FDA hasn't yet given that protection its unqualified approval.

Are you befuddled?

The way to clear your head is to remember that the male latex condom has the FDA's approval for use to protect against the virus that causes AIDS, and the female condom does not. Therefore, unless you are allergic to latex (see Chapter 8), the male latex condom should be the condom of choice.

If, for some reason—allergic reaction, plain old curiosity, whatever—you decide to use a female condom, your partner must not use a condom. If you decide to try it, you should stage a couple of rehearsals prior to putting it to use. And as of now, the female condom should, like the male condom, be used only once.

Temperature or age won't cause polyurethane to deteriorate, unlike latex. However, the same caveats apply to opening a female condom as its male counterpart. No frantic fingernails or teeth. Unroll it very, very gently so as not to tear it. The directions inside the box are clear, including easy-to-read diagrams. The female condom comes already lubricated.

Rub the outside of the pouch together to be sure the lubricant is evenly spread inside the pouch from the bottom to the top. Find a comfortable position. Put one foot on a chair or squat on a chair. Hold the pouch with the open end hanging down, then squeeze the ring you are holding and insert it until it is up past the pubic bone, where it fits comfortably. The outer ring covers the labia. The box the condoms come in contains extra tubes of lubricant in case you need it.

When you're finished, empty the condom into the toilet and knot it before you throw it away. Remember, the package recommends one-time use only. Ongoing research is exploring the safety of reuse, and the possibilities seem promising; UNAIDS and the World Health Organization are planning to convene a panel to consider reuse. But the manufacturer itself still doesn't favor washing and wearing.

In spite of its many drawbacks, the idea of the female condom is timely and legitimate. But in my market research, I found it practically nonexistent in pharmacies. In New York City I found one pharmacy that carried the female condom. But the pharmacist referred to it as Reality, a name that was phased out a couple of years ago, so maybe he doesn't do such a brisk business. Several others once carried the female condom but gave up because no customers came calling. Condomania, the condom supermarket in New York City, carries the female condom in their store and via mail order (Condomania.com, or 1–800–9–CON-DOM, 1–800–926–6366). The company reports that it sells extremely well.

Most pharmacies, it seems, aren't even aware of the female condom. Outside of New York City—upstate New York, out West, the Midwest—most pharmacists I contacted weren't tuned in to what I was talking about. (Be aware. I didn't do a broad or deep search; but I did enough to know that I would be stymied if I were personally searching for the FC and hadn't finally discovered it at Condomania.) And when you can find them, at almost $10.00 for a package of three, female condoms are also expensive, costing three times more than their male counterparts.

Ordinarily such spotty availability would bother me. I'd get indignant about second-class citizenship and the right to female empowerment, to choice. But right now female empowerment rests with the best protection available. And you've got it with the male latex condom.

CHAPTER TWELVE

NOT YOUR FATHER'S CONDOMS

47,000,000 infected, 0 cured

In the 1840s, the Goodyear Rubber Company mastered the technique of vulcanization (improving the strength and resiliency of rubber), and the mass production of condoms was off and running. Referred to early on as "rubbers," these condoms were straightforward, unadorned, and no-nonsense. The word "fun" wouldn't spring to mind looking at Mr. Goodyear's condoms.

In the 1930s, a more refined version of the rubber condom began to be marketed extensively. The raw material for latex condoms comes from *Hevea brasiliensis*, a tree grown in Malaysia. The latex condom is thinner than the original condom and thereby provides the wearer with more sensation. It also provides more protection than its precursor.

That was pretty much it for new condom thinking until the '90s, when a Japanese company, Okamoto, came along with some serious competition in the form of ultra-thin condoms. Their thinking was uncomplicated: safety that provided more pleasure.

An American company, Ansell, inspired by Japanese inventiveness, came up with an extensive line called Lifestyles, which introduced a condom with a domelike top that increased sensation. In response to the new competition, Trojan, the granddaddy of U.S. condom manufacturers, now 80 years old, started acting young again, with the introduction of its Pleasure condom, followed by Ultra-Pleasure.

The Trojan Company, owned by Carter-Wallace, controls 65 percent of the American condom market; in America its name is almost synonymous with the word condom.

An English firm, Durex, owned by SSL International, controls about 20 percent of worldwide condom sales.

Mayer, manufactured by London International Group, is highly regarded for its Kimono brand condoms. A specialty of this brand is its MAXX and MAXX PLUS, extra large and comfortably fitting sizes, and

Kimono Microthin, close to wearing nothing at all, so Mayer says.

As HIV/AIDS intruded itself into the bedrooms of the world, thus bestowing a new significance upon condoms, their manufacturers continued with more styles and more condom designs, designed to deliver thrills as well as safety.

In response to increasing evidence of latex allergies, other new non-latex condoms have recently been developed of a synthetic thermoplastic material. They have advantages over latex that include more and better transmission of body heat, thus providing more natural feeling; they are perhaps stronger than latex condoms, and they don't deteriorate under unfavorable storage conditions and are effective for prevention of pregnancy.

Several of these thermoplastic condoms are on the market now, but they do not, so far, protect against HIV/AIDS and are therefore useless in the battle against AIDS. But testing continues, and if they finally win FDA approval for protection against the transmission of the virus, they will be another weapon against the disease, particularly for all those who are allergic to latex.

Mass-produced condoms have changed radically—stunningly in fact—in response to their new, ever larger role in world health. There is considerable marketing inventiveness in this new generation of condoms. That inventiveness demonstrates an inherent common sense that faces up to the fact that sustained and pervasive condom use requires that condoms provide both safety and more sexual pleasure.

Wizard condom designers have come up with interesting, even stimulating new choices that don't compromise condoms' true purpose. Amid the sea of fascinating variations, however, beware of "novelty" condoms. They come packaged like lollipops or in plastic bubbles; they may look like sea anemones or rubber toys. Whatever they look like, they are, or should be, prominently labeled "novelty." Novelty means they *should not be used for intercourse*, because they offer no protection whatsoever. Regard them as a New Millennium flirting device. Give them as a gift, for a laugh, or as a hint of what's on your mind, but do not use them during intercourse, no matter what.

Besides the explosion in availability and choices, the main differences between your father's condoms and the condoms of the twenty-first century are not only thinness, discussed above, but also texture. Texture gives more traction, thus more pleasure, to both partners. Today's condoms have names like Rough Rider,

High Sensation, Intense Sensation, Pleasure Mesh, Erotica Vibra Ribbed, Shared Sensation, Night Light, Beyond Seven Studded (1350 studs, to be exact)—just for starters. The textures include ribs and studs (sometimes on the inside of the condom), textured xxxxxxxxxs. Sometimes the textures are pronounced, sometimes subtle.

There is a condom with a tiny amount of anesthetic, called Extended Pleasure. The anesthetic helps control the wearer's climax in order to better synchronize the climaxes of both partners. There's even a glow-in-the-dark condom that could go a long way toward preventing fumbling or, worse, a mistake. Think about it: a dark room and an intense condom need.

A condom called Inspiral has been getting high marks among buyers since 1998. It has curvy spirals that give it a loose-fitting, action-packed tip to create sexual friction and fun. An advanced version of Inspiral goes by the name Twisted Pleasure and sports a special thrilling twist at the closed end.

In early 2004 the ten top-selling condoms in the country were Durex Performax, Mayer Kimono MicroThin, Trojan Extended Pleasure and Pleasure Plus, Lifestyles Non-Lubricated with Mint, Trojan Supra, Mayer Kimono Sensation, Lifestyles Ultra Sensitive,

Durex Natural Feeling Non-Lubricated, and Durex Avanti Super Thin (non-latex). The business of condoms is so competitive that any or all of these brands could be bumped out of position at any time.

In South Africa, there's a new race-sensitive attitude to condom color. The government-sponsored condom dispensers (Condom Cans) have in the past been stocked with white condoms, but in response to black men's discomfort with white condoms the government now offers them in brown as well.

Condoms today come in many other colors as well (the colors won't rub off and don't cause any harm, and are pretty, if you care). Some come fragranced: strawberry, mint, orange, rose. And as for the ancient question, "Does size matter?" the answer is "yes" when it comes to condoms. Too small can be painful or even dangerous, since the condom may break. Too large and it may simply slide off and be useless.

Condom supermarkets provide a multitude of choices in an easygoing, anonymous atmosphere. You and your partner can shop together if you feel like it. Or stock up on your own for a rainy day. And, of course, the internet is a rich and convenient source for condoms—with plain brown wrapper anonymity.

The cost of this awesome little bit of technology

depends upon the package size. The basic cost, no matter how many ridges, studs, curlicues, xxxxxxs, colors, fragrances, is about $12.00 for twelve condoms.

Viewed against the price of not using condoms—illness and perhaps even death—that price is a big, fat bargain.

CHAPTER THIRTEEN

A CONDOM BY ANY
OTHER NAME . . .

47,000,000 infected, 0 cured

B efore you knew the word "condom," before you first stepped self-consciously up to a counter to buy one, you knew a slang word or two for this prophylactic device. The slang word did a pretty good job of clarifying what the condom was for. A good slang word does that. It will tell you something about the thing named. It will also impart some shock value. It is often emotionally charged.

You'll recognize some of these slang words for condoms—have no doubt uttered some of them yourself— but others will seem foreign to you, because many of them *are* foreign. The collection of words that follows is from Portugal, England, France, China, Australia, Germany, Hungary, Indonesia, Nigeria, the United States and South America. It comprises but a teeny, tiny drop in the world's reservoir of condom slang.

So, in case you're tired of calling a condom a condom, or are interested in broadening your vocabulary, here are a few options: American Letter, American Glove, Armor, Bag, Baggie, Balloon, Bishop, Buckskin, Bulletproof Vest, Cheater, Circular Protector, Cundum, Diving Suit, Dreadnought, Dobber, Eel-Skin, Envelope, Fearnought, Fish-Skin, F. L., French Letter, French Safe, Frenchy, Frog, Frog-Skin, Gentleman's Jerkin, The Goalie, Gossy, Jimmie Hatz, Italian Letter, Jo-Bag, Johnny, Johnny Bag, Love Glove, Lubie, Machine, Male Pessary, Naughty Bag, One-Piece Overcoat, Penis Guard, Penis Hat, Propho, Phallic Thimble, Port Said Garter, Raincoat, Rubber, Safe, Safety, Safety Sheath, Safety Tool, Scumbag, Sheath, Shower Cap, Spanish Letter, Skin, Specialty, Spitfire, Venus Shirt, Willie Warmer, Zarape.

CHAPTER FOURTEEN

LAST (BUT NOT LEAST) WORDS

47,000,000 infected, 0 cured

I n case you haven't read this book but would like to absorb its message fast, here's what you should know, in twelve simple, life-saving messages.

1. The male latex condom is the best protection against sexual transmission of HIV/AIDS to date (excluding abstinence) that medicine has to offer.

2. All adults are responsible for their own protection from HIV/AIDS. (There are certain populations that require special protection, e.g., unborn babies, adolescents, prisoners, and the mentally retarded.)

3. Alcohol, marijuana, crystal methamphetamine, the drug colloquially known as special K, and a very long

list of other drugs should be avoided prior to having sex. They impair one's ability to think or act responsibly.

4. Approximately 1.2 million persons in the United States are infected with HIV. Of these, approximately one quarter are unaware of their status. We all must bear the responsibility for this tragedy.

5. Even a person bearing a legitimate negative laboratory report can still be HIV-positive. Tennis legend Arthur Ashe, who died of AIDS-related pneumonia, reportedly became infected when he received blood that had tested negative for HIV before the transfusion. The transfusion took place during the "window period," when it was too soon for the test to show the antibodies.

6. Condoms must be used consistently, 100 percent of the time, and correctly 100 percent of the time to provide maximum protection.

7. It is far better to offend your partner by demanding (negotiating) condom use than to trust him and risk becoming infected. One of the issues lied about most frequently is with whom one has or has not had sex. And check out Chapter 4 for information about the "Down Lows" and their contribution to the AIDS pandemic.

8. The "morning-after treatment" (see Glossary) for high-risk sexual behavior is not effective in preventing HIV. The male latex condom is effective.

9. Waiting for the vaccine to prevent HIV? It's likely to be a long wait. Besides, vaccines are available to prevent many diseases but are not always used when appropriate. For example, the vaccine for hepatitis B is recommended and available to all who need it, yet is rarely used by those who need it most. So, even if a vaccine is someday developed, there are many who would not take advantage of it, especially as it would probably need to be repeated yearly.

10. Female polyurethane condoms are now available. However, the relatively short time they have been available makes conclusions about their safety and acceptability pale by comparison to the gold standard—the male latex condom. See Chapter 10.

11. "Learning to love yourself is the greatest love of all" according to a famous Whitney Houston song. When you masturbate, you can have sex without a condom.

12. There are HIV-positive people who don't value their lives. "Someone gave it to me. I'm going to give it to as many people as possible." Beware of those bearing the virus. Make sure they keep it to them-

selves. "Undetectable" does not mean the person is not infectious; one must still use condoms.

GLOSSARY

Abstinence

When used in a sexual context, choosing not to indulge in sex. It is now commonly used to refer to denying oneself intercourse, while indulging in other sexual acts, e.g., oral sex.

AIDS

Acquired Immunodeficiency Syndrome, the disease state caused by HIV (Human Immunodeficiency Virus). There are 21 AIDS-defining conditions listed by the CDC. The one most commonly referred to by most lay people is the CD4 cell count.

Barebacking

A term used to describe the practice of having anal sex without a condom.

Condom fatigue

A term used to describe weariness of the condom health message ("tired of hearing about them, even more tired of using them").

Condom Types and Their Properties

Condom Types	Properties
Latex	Barrier protection against HIV, STDs, and pregnancy FDA-approved
Polyurethane	Efficacy in preventing HIV transmission likely to be similar to latex condoms (only a limited number of efficacy studies to date) Not yet approved by the FDA in preventing transmission of HIV More expensive Alternative for latex allergy Conducts heat and therefore improves sensitivity
Female	Allows for direct control by the woman Covers both internal and external genitalia Efficacy in preventing HIV transmission estimated to be equivalent to, or slightly less than, the male condom (limited number of studies regarding efficacy to date) Not approved by the FDA
Lambskin	Does not protect against HIV transmission (microscopic pores allow transfer of HIV virions but not bacterial STD pathogens) Effective against pregnancy
Styrene ethylene butylene styrene (SEBS)	Alternative for latex allergy Efficacy in preventing HIV transmission inadequately studied

Condom

A sheath made of one of several materials (latex, lamb-skin, polyurethane) worn over the penis to prevent sexually transmitted diseases and pregnancy. A female condom also exists, and the development of a rectal condom is in the works.

"Down low"

Also called the DL and "Tarzan by day, Jane by night." The practice of men who secretly have sex with men but do not self-identify as bisexual. Their homosexual activities are kept secret from friends, associates, and their unsuspecting female partners. *No More Secrets, No More Lies*, by J. L. King, is a recent documentary about the "down low" lifestyle.

Glory holes

Holes in walls usually found in bathhouses and toilet partitions in sex clubs and bars that permit anonymous sex. The holes are just large enough to permit the penis to pass through the partition and into the mouth or rectum of an unknown recipient on the other side.

HIV

The virus that causes AIDS. There are two types. The most common type in the United States is Type 1. Type 2 comes from West Africa.

"Morning-after pill"

Antiretrovirals (name for medications used to treat HIV/AIDS) taken the morning after risky sexual behavior in the mistaken belief that the medication will prevent HIV. The practice is based on the contraceptive prevention model, which has been tested and is safe, unlike taking antiretrovirals the morning after.

Prophylactic

Another common name for condom, denoting its purpose.

Rubber

Early name for condom; still used.

Trojans

A brand name of the first large producer of condoms, now used in much the same way as "Xerox" and "Kleenex" are used to denote copiers and facial tissue.

Undetectable

Following a blood test called a viral load, a statement that denotes that HIV was not detected in a person know to be HIV-positive. Undetectable does not mean cured; measurement in vaginal secretions or semen would still show the presence of the virus.

Window period

The time delay from the time of exposure to the time one tests positive for HIV. With newer tests, that period can be as short as 14 days. According to an article in one of the most reliable medical journals (*American Journal of Medicine*) virtually everyone exposed to HIV converts by six months.

RESOURCES

There is a Department of Health where you live. Every state capital, and most major cities, have one. Each is able to give advice about local HIV counseling, testing and treatment sites. The National Association of Community Health Centers (NACHC) represents Federally Qualified Community Health Centers in the 50 states, Puerto Rico and the Virgin Islands through their Primary Care Associations (PCAs). You can find the information for your state at www.nachc.com.

WEBSITES
Where to order condoms
www.condom.com
www.condomania.com
www.condomcorner.com
www.condomdepot.com
www.CondomExpress.com
www.craigsweb.com/condom4.htm
www.ShopInSecret.com

Where to Get Help

AIDS Hotline for teens	1-800-TALK-HIV 1-800-825-5448 www.iwannaknow.org
Gay Men's Health Crisis (GMHC)	1-800-243-7692 www.gmhc.org
Health Watch	1-877-40-HEALTH www.hwatch.org
HIV/AIDS Treatment Information Service	1-800-448-0440
National AIDS Hotline	1-800-342-2437 (English) 1-800-344-7432 (Spanish)
National Hope Line (formerly called Suicide Line)	1-800-784-2433
National Sexually Transmitted Disease/ AIDS Hotline	1-800-227-8922
National AIDS Hotline Telephone-Typewriter Service	1-800-243-7889 www.ashastd.org/nah/tty.html
National Herpes Hotline	1-800-230-6039

SUGGESTED READINGS

ARTICLES

The following is a catalog of articles pertinent to the subject of this book. Be aware that, unlike books listed in a traditional bibliography, web sites tend to have short lifespans. The articles cited may have passed out of cyberspace by the time this book has reached you.

"Approved with restrictive labeling—the Reality Female Condom," Food and Drug Administration, April 26, 1993, http://www.fda.gov/bbs/topics/NEWS/NEW00360.html.

Beresford, Belinda, "Brown condoms for clever dicks: The government believes black men find white condoms off-putting." *Daily Mail and Guardian* (Johannesburg), September 4, 2004, http://www.aegis.com/news/dmg/2000/MG000901.html.

Davies, Chris, MEP, Liberal Democrat Member of the European Parliament for the North West of England, "North West MEP urges Catholics to question local priests," December 9, 2003, http://www.chrisdaviesmep.org.uk/news/2003/December/north_west_mep_urges_catholics_to_question_local_priests.htm.

Dotinga, Randy, "Female condom has its limits," HealthScout-News, March 4, 2003, http://www.hon.ch/News/HSN/511891.html.

"FC instructions and tips for use," Mayer Labs, Socially Responsible Healthcare, http://www.mayerlabs.com/consumer/products/fcfemaleinstruct.asp.

"The female condom: Controlled by women," *Network*, Vol. 16, No. 1, Family Health International, September 1995, http://www.fhi.org/en/RH/Pubs/Network/v16_1/nt16110.htm.

Frezieres RG, Walsh TL, Nelson AL, Clark VA, Coulson AH, "Breakage and acceptability of a polyeurethane condom: A randomized, controlled study," *Family Planning Perspectives*, March–April 1998, 73–8, http://www.ncbi.nlm.nih.gov/entrez/query.fcgi?db=Pmc.

Gates, Melinda French, "AIDS and India," *Seattle Times*, April 11, 2004, http://archives.seattletimes.nwsource.com/cgi-bin/texis.cgi/web/vortex/display?slug=gates11&date=20040411.

Glickman, Adam, "The condom promised land," July 13, 2004,
    http://www.freewebs.com/datingpages/condoms.htm.

Hooper, Ernest, "Black men on the 'down low' and AIDS are scary
    trends," *St. Petersburg Times*, April 15, 2004,
    http://pqasb.pqarchiver.com/sptimes/618367641.html?MAC=0c
    315ce2d6e6ad992f1c9b30c3f24475&did=618367641&FMT=FTT

James, John S., "Nonoxynol-9 dangers: Health experts warn
    against rectal use," *AIDS Treatment News*, October 18, 2002,
    http://www.findarticles.com/p/articles/mi_m0HSW/is_384/ai_
    93657693.

Kristof, Nicholas D., "Don't tell the Pope," *The New York Times*,
    November 26, 2003,
        http://www.phrusa.org/campaigns/aids/news112603_NYT.html.

Kristof, Nicholas D., "The secret war on condoms," *The New York
    Times*, January 10, 2003,
        http://www.natap.org/2003/Jan/011403_7.htm.

Neurenberg, Rebecca, "Condoms in correctional settings," *HEPP
    News*, Vol. 5, Issue 1, January 2002,
        http://www.thebody.com/hepp/jan02/spotlight.html.

"Prescription transfers and information," Birth Control Pill.net,
    http://www.birth-control-pill.net/condoms.php.

"Protect yourself! Respect yourself!" UAHIV Info Prevention,
http://www.albany.edu/sph/AIDS/prevention_1.html.

"The role of condoms in preventing HIV infection and other sexually transmitted diseases," CDC National Aids Hotline Train-
ing Bulletin #23, Centers for Disease Control and Prevention,
February 22, 1993,
http://www.aegis.com/pubs/Cdc_Fact_Sheets/1993/CDC9312
5.html.

"So little time . . . An AIDS/HIV History,"
http://www.aegis.com/topics/timeline/default.asp.

"Special Focus: Condoms and HIV/AIDS," RHO Reproductive
Health Outlook, updated 2004,
http://www.rho.org/html/hiv_aids_special_focus-condoms.htm.

"Strategies for preventing HIV in women: How can women protect themselves?" July 1997, Centers for Disease Control and
Prevention,
http://www.thebody.com/cdc/women/strategy4.html.

"Top 10 condoms," CondomUSA.com,
http://www.condomusa.com/4editor.asp.

Wetzstein, Cheryl, " 'Condom fatigue' on increase," *The Washington Times*, November 8, 2002,
http://www.washingtontimes.com.

"Your tax dollars are being wasted ruining citizens' lives instead of fighting real crime," Decriminalize Prostitution Now Coalition, http://www.sexwork.com/coalition/whatcountrieslegal.html.

BOOKS

The following titles are recommended for further reading.

Ackerman, Diane, 1990. *A Natural History of the Senses.* New York: Random House.

Altman, Dennis, 2001. *Global Sex.* Chicago: University of Chicago Press.

Chapple, Steve, and David Talbot, 1989. *Burning Desires: Sex in America: A Report from the Field.* New York: Doubleday.

Delacoste, Frédérique Y, and Priscilla Alexander, editors, 1987. *Sex Work: Writings by Women in the Sex Industry.* San Francisco: Cleis Press.

Drinka, George Frederick, MD, 1984. *The Birth of Neurosis, Myth, Malady, and the Victorians.* New York: Simon and Schuster.

Fisher, Helen E., 1992. *Anatomy of Love: The Natural History of Monogamy, Adultery, and Divorce.* New York: W.W. Norton.

Foucault, Michel, 1978. *The History of Sexuality.* New York: Pantheon Books.

Gay, Peter, 2002. *Schnitzler's Century: The Making of Middle Class Culture, 1815–1914.* New York: W.W. Norton.

Hite, Shere, 1987. *The Hite Report: Women in Love: A Cultural Revolution in Progress.* New York: Alfred A. Knopf.

Partridge, Eric, and Paul Beale, editors, 1990. *Partridge's Concise Dictionary of Slang and Unconventional English.* Old Tappan, NJ: John Wiley & Sons Inc.

Pheterson, Gail, editor, 1989. *A Vindication of the Rights of Whores.* Emeryville, CA: The Seal Press.

Showalter, Elaine, 1990. *Sexual Anarchy: Gender and Culture at the Fin de Siècle.* New York: Viking Press.